MARSH TACKY HORSE

The Complete Handbook On How To Raising And Caring For Marsh Tacky Horse

CHAD BRUNO

Table of Contents

Introductory

Originally from the marshy areas of South Carolina's Atlantic coast, the Marsh Tacky horse breed is now found all over the world. The word "tacky," which originally referred to a common or unremarkable horse, is where the name "Marsh Tacky" comes from. These horses are known for their resilience, adaptability, and hardiness in the challenging marshy environments they inhabit.

Marsh Tackies range in size from about 13 to 15 hands (52 to 60 inches) in height. They come in various colors, although solid colors such as bay, black, and gray are common. These horses have a special talent for finding their way through South Carolina's wetlands and along the coast. Their stamina and strength made them useful for herding cattle, hunting, and transporting goods across difficult terrain.

Changes in land use and a decline in the breed's popularity in recent years have both threatened the survival of Marsh Tackies. Because of their historical and cultural significance to the state of South Carolina, conservation efforts have

been made to protect this rare
horse breed.

CHAPTER ONE
Character and Conduct

Like horses of any breed, Marsh Tacky horses can exhibit a wide range of personalities and behaviors. There are, however, some defining characteristics and traits shared by dogs of this breed in general:

1. Marsh Tackies are renowned for their work ethic and versatility, and for good reason. They have a long history of service in arduous conditions, and they are willing workers.

2. Ability to learn quickly and efficiently is a common compliment to these horses' intelligence. They are flexible and resourceful, able to adjust to new situations with ease.

3. Marsh Tackies are known for their steady temperament and low activity levels. They have a more even temperament and are less easily startled than other dog breeds. Their demeanor lends itself well to duties that call for consistency.

4. Similar to other horses, Marsh Tackies enjoy company. Horses and humans alike benefit greatly from social interaction. Dogs have a high propensity for developing close relationships with their owners, making them relatively simple to train.

5. Alert and Curious: Marsh Tackies are typically alert and curious about their surroundings. This can be an advantage in their native environments, where they need to navigate challenging terrain and potentially encounter wildlife.

6. Due to their long history of surviving in harsh conditions, these horses have become somewhat self-sufficient. They usually have to rely on themselves and their own wits.

7. Stamina and endurance are hallmarks of Marsh Tackies. They are able to travel great distances and to toil for long periods of time without becoming fatigued.

It's important to remember that each horse is an individual, and that training, socialization, and handling can all have an effect on a horse's behavior. Marsh Tackies, like dogs of any breed, need to be trained and cared for properly to ensure they behave well and trust their owners or handlers. The health and success of your dog's training depends on your familiarity with the breed's unique requirements and personality quirks.

Need for Safe Place to Stay

Like all other horse breeds, Marsh Tackys need shelter that is appropriate for the local climate and environment. They have adapted to the harsh conditions of their native habitat in the marshy regions of South Carolina, where summers are hot and humid and winters are mild. Some things to keep in mind when building a stable for Marsh Tacky horses:

1. Shelter from the elements: heavy rain, strong winds, and intense heat can all be avoided inside a well-ventilated stable or barn. Make sure there is adequate drainage to

prevent water from pooling and the structure is stable and secure.

2. Paddocks or Pastures: Horses need access to outdoor areas for exercise and grazing. Ensure that pastures or paddocks are securely fenced to keep the horses safe and to prevent them from wandering into unsafe areas.

3. In extremely hot and sunny climates, shade is a necessity. Although trees' natural shading is helpful, if it isn't enough, you may want to build shade structures or put up run-in sheds in your pastures.

4. Air Quality Maintenance and Contamination Prevention Adequate ventilation is essential to prevent the buildup of harmful fumes from manure and to maintain air quality within the stable or barn.

5. Bedding: Make sure the stalls have soft bedding like straw or shavings. This helps keep the horses dry, clean, and comfortable.

6. Make sure there's a good supply of clean water close by the shelter or pasture. Horses require a significant amount of water daily to stay hydrated.

7. Feeding Area: If you feed your Marsh Tacky horses in a stable or barn, designate a specific feeding area to prevent food aggression and keep the space clean.

8. Security: Ensure that the shelter is secure to protect the horses from predators and to prevent them from escaping. Gates and doors should be in good working condition.

9. Maintenance: Regular maintenance is important to keep the shelter safe and functional. Check for structural integrity, repair any damage promptly, and keep the area clean to prevent health issues.

10. Climate Considerations: Depending on the climate in your region, you may need to take additional steps to protect Marsh Tacky horses from extreme cold or heat. This could include heated water sources in winter or fans and cooling systems in hot weather.

It's important to adapt the shelter and care of Marsh Tacky horses to the specific conditions of your location. Consult with local equine experts or veterinarians for guidance on providing appropriate shelter and care for your horses based on your regional climate and environmental factors.

CHAPTER TWO

Dietary Needs of Marsh Tackies

The dietary needs of Marsh Tacky horses are similar to those of most other horse breeds, with some considerations based on the individual horse's age, activity level, and health. Here are some general guidelines for the dietary needs of Marsh Tacky horses:

1. Forage (Grass and Hay): The foundation of a horse's diet should be high-quality forage. In their native marshy environments, Marsh Tackies would have grazed on a variety of grasses and plants. Provide access to good pasture for grazing, and if pasture quality is inadequate, supplement with good-quality hay. The type of hay should be chosen based on the nutritional needs of the horse, the available options, and any specific health considerations.

2. Water: Clean, fresh water should always be available to Marsh Tacky horses. Horses can drink a significant amount of water, and proper hydration is crucial for their overall health.

3. Concentrates (Grain): The amount and type of concentrates (grain) you feed your Marsh Tacky will depend on their individual needs. Concentrates are typically used to provide additional energy and nutrients. Young, growing horses, pregnant or lactating mares, and horses in heavy work may require more concentrates. However, many Marsh Tackies can maintain their health and energy levels on forage alone.

4. Minerals and Supplements: Depending on the quality of the forage and the specific needs of the horse, you may need to provide mineral supplements. Consult with a veterinarian or equine nutritionist to determine if any specific minerals or supplements are necessary.

5. Avoid Overfeeding: Overfeeding can lead to obesity and related health problems in horses. Ensure that you are providing the right amount of food for the horse's activity level and metabolic needs. Monitor the horse's body condition to make adjustments as needed.

6. Regular Feeding Schedule: Horses thrive on a consistent feeding schedule. They should be fed at the same times each day, with access to forage throughout the day.

7. Consult with a Veterinarian or Nutritionist: It's a good idea to consult with a veterinarian or equine nutritionist to create a customized feeding plan for your Marsh Tacky horses. They can help you assess the specific nutritional needs of your horses and make recommendations accordingly.

8. Health Considerations: Take into account any health conditions or special dietary requirements of your individual horses. For example, older horses or those with metabolic issues may require specialized diets.

Remember that the dietary needs of Marsh Tacky horses can vary based on factors such as age, activity level, climate, and overall health. Regular monitoring of your horses' body condition and consulting with equine professionals will help ensure that their dietary requirements are met for optimal health and performance.

Healthcare and Veterinary Care

Proper healthcare and veterinary care are essential for keeping Marsh Tacky horses healthy and ensuring their well-being. Here are some important aspects to consider:

1. Regular Veterinary Checkups:
Just like any other horse breed, Marsh Tackies should have regular veterinary checkups. These checkups can help identify and address potential health issues early, ensuring your horses stay in good health.

2. Vaccinations: Consult with your veterinarian to establish a vaccination schedule that is appropriate for your region and the specific health risks your horses may face. Vaccinations can protect them from diseases like tetanus, Eastern and Western equine encephalitis, and West Nile virus.

3. Dental Care: Horses, including Marsh Tackies, have teeth that continually grow, and dental issues can affect their health and nutrition. Regular dental checkups and floating (filing down sharp points and uneven surfaces) are essential for maintaining their oral health.

4. Parasite Control: Regular deworming is crucial to control internal parasites. Work with your veterinarian to develop a deworming schedule tailored to your horses' needs and the local parasite prevalence.

5. Hoof Care: Regular hoof care, including trimming and shoeing, is essential to maintain healthy hooves and prevent lameness. The frequency of trimming and shoeing will depend on the individual horse's needs and activity level.

6. Nutritional Assessment: Consult with an equine nutritionist or your veterinarian to ensure your horses are receiving a balanced diet appropriate for their age, activity level, and any specific health concerns.

7. Emergency Care Plan: Have an emergency care plan in place in case your Marsh Tacky horses experience a medical crisis. This should include contact information for your veterinarian and the nearest equine hospital or clinic.

8. Preventative Care: Take preventative measures to reduce the risk of injuries and illnesses. This can include providing safe fencing and housing, maintaining a clean and well-ventilated environment, and practicing good biosecurity to prevent the spread of diseases.

9. Training and Handling: Ensure that your horses are properly trained and handled to reduce stress during veterinary examinations and treatments. A well-mannered horse is safer for both the animal and the healthcare providers.

10. Records and Documentation: Keep accurate records of your horses' health, vaccinations, deworming, dental care, and any medical treatments. This information is valuable for tracking their healthcare history and making informed decisions.

11. Education and Resources: Stay informed about the latest advances in equine healthcare and veterinary practices. Attend workshops, seminars, and training programs to enhance your knowledge and skills in caring for Marsh Tacky horses.

Remember that individual horses may have unique healthcare needs, so working closely with a qualified equine veterinarian is crucial for providing the best care for your Marsh Tacky horses. Tailoring healthcare and veterinary care to the specific needs of each horse is essential for their long-term health and well-being.

CHAPTER THREE
Training and Handling

Training and handling Marsh Tacky horses, like any horse breed, requires patience, consistency, and a good understanding of equine behavior. Here are some guidelines for training and handling these horses:

1. Establish Trust: Building trust is the foundation of any successful training program. Spend time with your horse, petting and grooming them to establish a bond. Horses are more likely to respond positively to a handler they trust.

2. Start Early: Begin training when the horse is young, if possible. Younger horses tend to be more adaptable and willing to learn. However, older horses can also be trained, but it may take more time and patience.

3. Use Positive Reinforcement: Reward good behavior with praise, treats, or pats. Positive reinforcement is an effective way to motivate horses and encourage them to repeat desired behaviors.

4. Consistency: Be consistent in your cues, commands, and expectations. Horses thrive on routine and predictability.

Inconsistent handling can confuse and stress them.

5. Groundwork: Groundwork is an important part of horse training. Teaching your horse to lead, lunge, and respond to cues from the ground will establish a solid foundation for riding and other activities.

6. Basic Obedience: Teach your horse basic commands like "walk," "trot," "halt," and "back up." Make sure they respond to these cues reliably before moving on to more advanced training.

7. Desensitization: Expose your horse to various sights, sounds, and objects to desensitize them to potential sources of fear. Gradual exposure and positive reinforcement can help them become less reactive.

8. Riding Training: If you plan to ride your Marsh Tacky, introduce the horse to a saddle, bridle, and rider gradually. Start with groundwork to build confidence and then proceed to mounting and riding in a safe, controlled **environment.**

9. Seek Professional Help: If you're not experienced in horse training or encounter behavioral challenges that you're unsure how to address, it's a good idea to seek the assistance of a professional horse trainer. They can provide valuable guidance and training techniques.

10. Be Patient: Training can be a slow and gradual process. Horses may need time to understand and respond to new commands. Patience and a calm demeanor are essential.

11. Safety: Prioritize safety for both you and the horse. Wear appropriate safety gear, and avoid putting yourself in situations that could lead to injury. Know your horse's body language and be aware of potential signs of stress or discomfort.

12. Social Interaction: Horses are social animals, and they benefit from interaction with other horses. Provide opportunities for your Marsh Tacky to socialize with other equines, as this can contribute to their overall well-being.

13. Regular Exercise: Regular exercise and turnout are essential for a horse's physical and mental well-being. Ensure your Marsh Tacky gets enough time for grazing and movement.

Remember that every horse is an individual with its own personality and learning pace. Tailor your training approach to the specific needs and temperament of your Marsh Tacky, and be open to adjusting your methods as necessary to achieve the desired results while ensuring the horse's well-being and comfort.

Breeding and Reproduction

Breeding and reproduction in Marsh Tacky horses, like in any horse breed, involves careful planning, health considerations, and knowledge of equine reproductive processes. Here are some key points to consider when it comes to breeding and reproduction in Marsh Tackies:

1. Breeding Goals: Determine your breeding goals. Are you breeding for preservation and promotion of the breed, for specific traits, or for specific purposes like riding, working, or showing? Understanding your goals will help guide your breeding decisions.

2. Selecting Breeding Stock: Choose healthy, genetically sound, and well-tempered Marsh Tacky horses as breeding stock. Consider their conformation, temperament, and any relevant performance or lineage factors.

3. Health Assessment: Prior to breeding, both the mare and stallion should undergo a thorough veterinary examination to ensure they are in good health and free from reproductive issues. Vaccinations and deworming should be up to date.

4. Timing of Breeding: Determine the optimal time for breeding. Most mares have a natural breeding season during the spring and summer, but artificial insemination allows for year-round breeding. Consult with a veterinarian or equine reproduction specialist for guidance on timing.

5. Stallion Selection: If using natural breeding, choose a suitable stallion. If using artificial insemination, collect and store semen from a chosen stallion, or select a stallion from a breeding facility.

6. Mare Care: Care for the mare during pregnancy. This includes proper nutrition, regular exercise, and veterinary care to monitor her health and the health of the developing foal.

7. Foaling Preparations: Prepare for the foaling process. This includes creating a clean, safe foaling environment and having the necessary supplies on hand.

8. Post-Foaling Care: After foaling, provide appropriate care for the mare and foal. Monitor the foal's health, make sure it nurses successfully, and ensure that the mare recovers well from the birth.

9. Weaning: Decide on the appropriate time for weaning the foal. Weaning typically occurs around 4 to 6 months of age, but the timing can vary based on individual circumstances.

10. Registration: If you're breeding Marsh Tackies for breed preservation, ensure that your foals are registered with the appropriate breed registry to maintain their pedigree records.

11. Educational Resources: Stay informed about the latest in equine reproduction and breeding practices. Attending workshops and seeking advice from experienced breeders and veterinarians can be helpful.

12. Ethical Considerations: Ensure that your breeding practices align with ethical and responsible breeding principles. Avoid overbreeding and contribute positively to the breed's conservation and development.

Remember that breeding and reproduction require a commitment of time, resources, and knowledge. It's important to approach breeding with a clear understanding of your goals and responsibilities, and to prioritize the health and well-being of the horses involved. Consulting with experienced breeders and veterinarians is highly recommended when embarking on a breeding program with Marsh Tacky horses or any other breed.

Conclusion

Marsh Tacky horses are a unique and hardy breed known for their adaptability and resilience in challenging marshy environments. Proper care and management are essential to ensure the health and well-being of these horses. This includes providing suitable shelter, balanced nutrition, regular veterinary care, and thoughtful training and handling.

Breeding and reproduction in Marsh Tackies should be approached with careful planning, taking into account breeding goals, the health of the breeding stock, and ethical considerations. Preservation of the breed's genetic heritage and promotion of desirable traits are important aspects of responsible breeding.

Overall, Marsh Tacky horses are not only a valuable part of South Carolina's cultural heritage but also a breed with qualities that make them suitable for various equestrian pursuits, from working on the land to recreational riding. Whether you're a breeder, owner, or enthusiast, understanding the unique characteristics and needs of Marsh Tacky horses is essential for their conservation and responsible management.

THE END

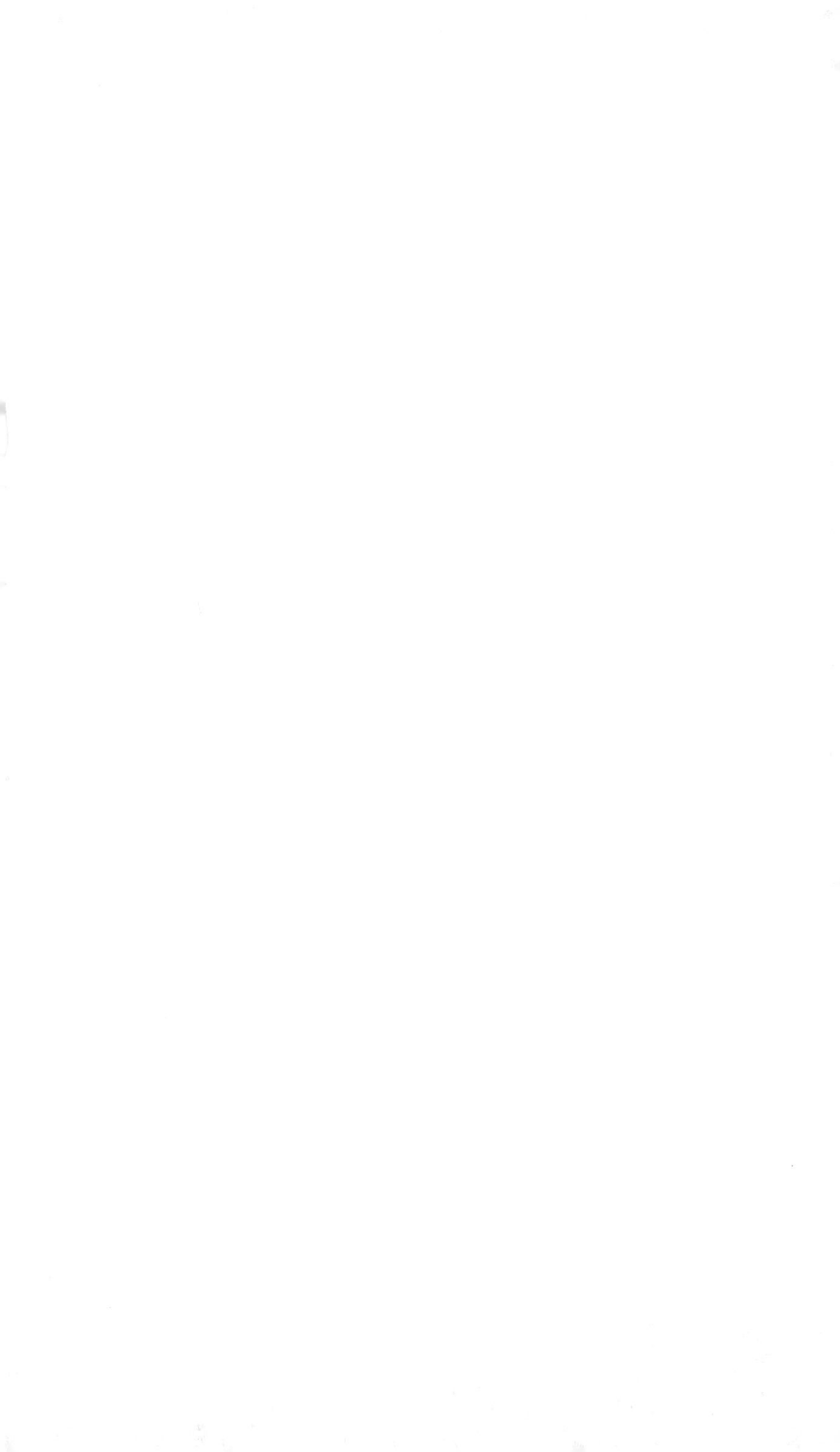

www.ingramcontent.com/pod-product-compliance
Lightning Source LLC
Chambersburg PA
CBHW072251310526
45795CB00011B/946